The Clothes of the Cut

-a history of canal costume

by

Avril Lansdell

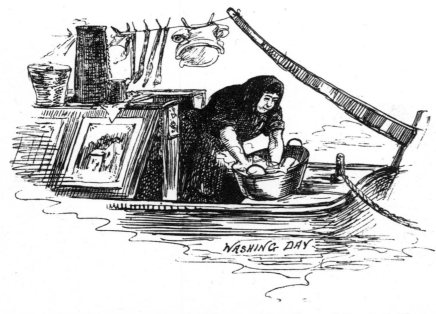

One of a series of sketches '*Life on Canal Boats*' from the Illustrated Sporting and Dramatic News 1884

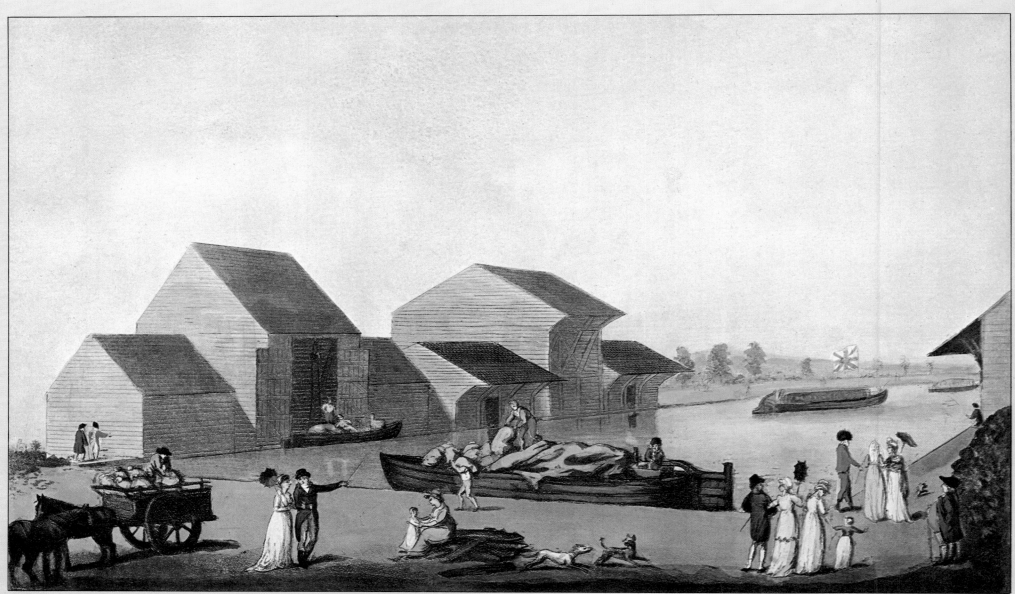

A view of the Basin of the Grand Junction Canal, Paddington 1801

Contents

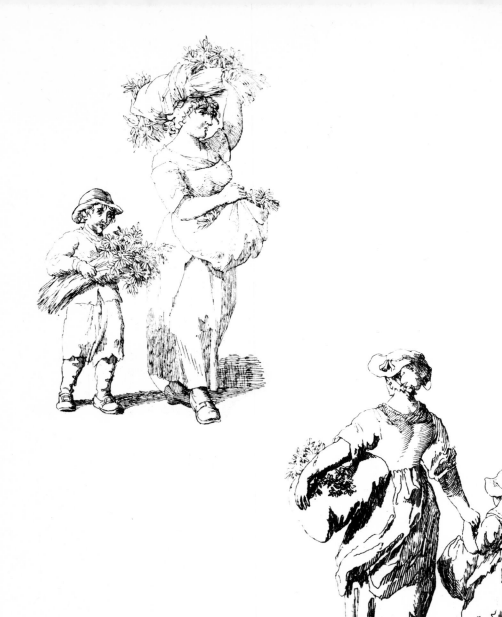

Acknowledgements

The author would like to thank the following for their help in contributing information and answering questions and letters

R. J. Hutchings — Waterways Museum, Stoke Bruerne
John Scholes, F.M.A. — Museum of British Transport
George Shearer, A.M.A. — Worcester County Museum
Dr D. E. Owen, F.M.A. — Manchester Museum
The Librarian — The English Folk Song and Dance Society
John Goodchild — Cusworth Hall Museum, Doncaster
Pamela Clabburn — Strangers' Hall Museum, Norwich

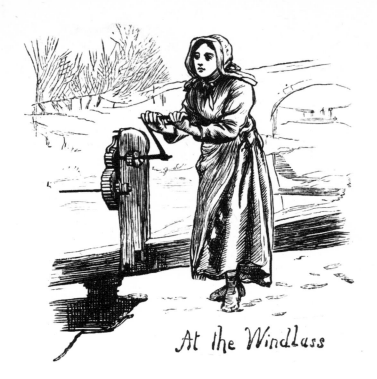

At the Windlass

Illustration of boatwoman from an 1875 edition of '*The Graphic*'.

Introduction

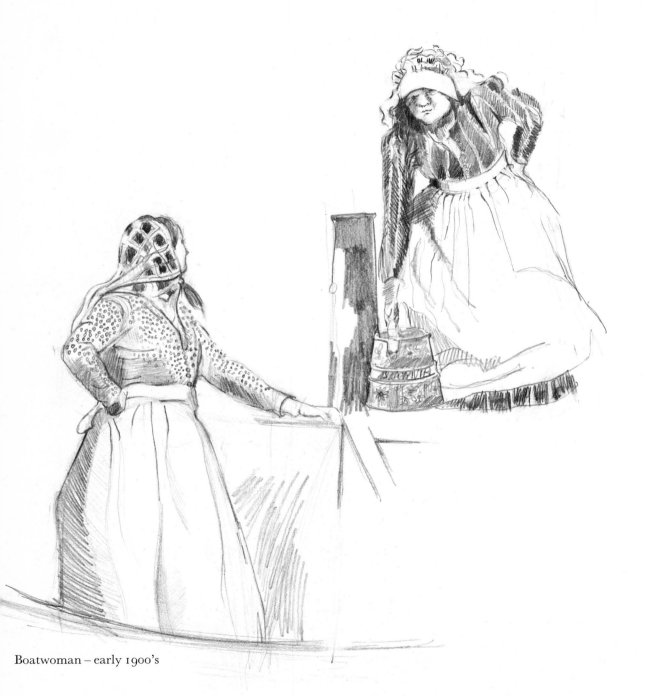

Boatwoman – early 1900's

Avril Lansdell, A.M.A., has been curator of Weybridge Museum since 1968 and is the author of *The Wey Navigation (A Tale of Troubled Waters)*. She became interested in canal costume when she took a museum diploma in folk life and local history. Her thesis on the surviving occupational costume in the museums of England and Wales involved visits to the Waterways Museum at Stoke Bruerne to study items of canal clothing. Although Avril Lansdell became associated with canals purely from a costume point of view, her interest in the subject and her visits to the Waterways Museum have turned her into an enthusiast.

In the late 1940's Avril Lansdell studied the history of costume and design at art school. After her marriage she did freelance work on theatrical costumes, and lectured in South London on stage costume and production on behalf of the Kingston Council of Churches. Professional painting followed after her children were born and four exhibitions of her work were held, two in London. She also lectured on the history of costume, and joined the Weybridge Museum in 1966 as costume and display assistant.

In 1970, two years after becoming curator of the museum, she examined canal costumes at Manchester, Norwich and Stoke Bruerne when studying occupational costume of all types for her thesis. Richard Hutchings had recently become curator at Stoke Bruerne. She gave him advice on how to clean the canal clothes there and classified and dated them. Considerable public interest followed and the need arose for an expert publication, which would contribute both to the history of costume and to the history of the waterways;—thus evolved *Clothes of the Cut*.

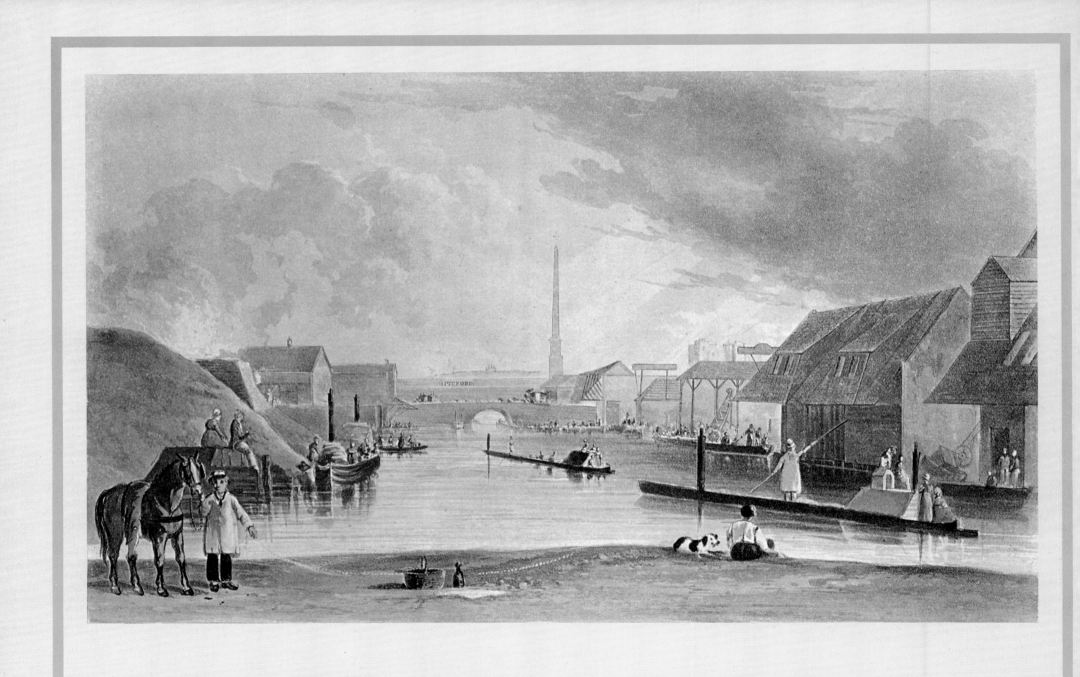

The City Basin, Regent's Canal, early 1800's

1. Beginnings

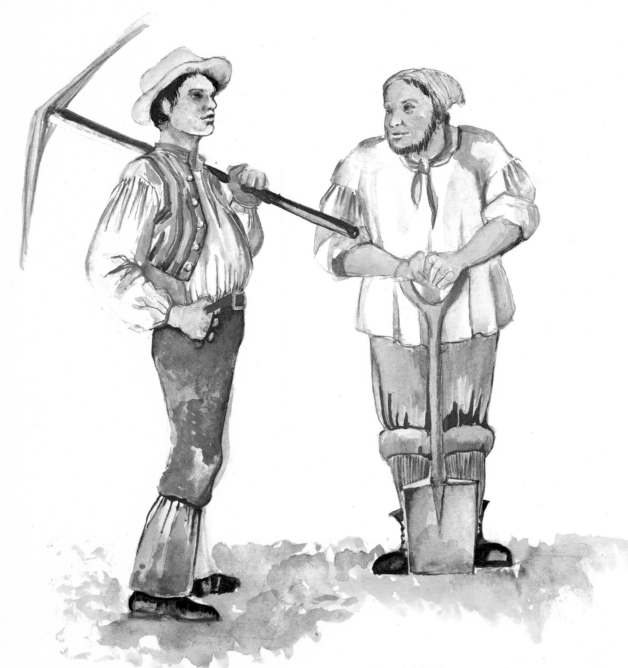

Navvies, based on drawings that appeared in '*Punch*' 1814 (left) and 1846 (right)

Between 1760 and 1840 the landscape of England, particularly that of the Midlands, was changed by the building of the canals. They were part of the industrial revolution and their existence contributed very substantially to the growing prestige and prosperity of middle-class England. Yet this middle-class prosperity which was to lead Napoleon to describe England as a 'nation of shopkeepers' was the result of co-operation between two other classes of people, the aristocrats and the thousands of unknown men and women who dug the canals and manned the boats which carried goods along those inland waterways. The deeds of the 3rd Duke of Bridgewater, Francis Egerton, engineers such as Brindley and Telford, manufacturers such as Spode and Wedgwood are well known but their ideas and aspirations would have been of no use without the work of the 'navvies' and boatmen whose colourful clothes and distinctive lives are part of the background of English industrial history.

The generations of men known as 'navvies', who dug canals and fifty years later moved on to lay railway tracks, were a community strong enough to develop their own way of life. They did not stay long enough in any one place to influence those living there, and, like gypsies, were looked on as both disruptive and romantic outsiders. The name 'navvy' derived from their original work on the canals where they were known as 'navigators'. Because it was not easy for a man to work as a navvy and maintain a family, the camps which housed these wandering workmen included women and children who often lived in extremely insanitary conditions and in dire poverty. Some of these women were wives according to the law of the land, but many more were wives according to the ceremonies (if any) which were evolved by the navvies themselves who felt in little need of the established church. Because men far outnumbered women, reports and illustrations of them do not tell us what these women wore, but the men were colourful and distinctive. In the eighteenth century they wore breeches, shirts, waistcoats and stocking caps. Some reports of the navvies say that they wore smocks, but their 'smocks' are more likely to have been their shirts worn outside their breeches when they were not wearing waistcoats. Eighteenth century shirts were very wide; without a waistcoat to hold them in place they would soon pull free of breeches when the wearer was working strenuously. The most important item of a navvy's equipment and clothing was his pair of boots. These were far heavier and stronger than boots worn by other workers. The bottoms of the canals, once they were dug, had to be lined with a thick layer of clay to prevent water draining away. Preparation of the clay was called 'puddling'. A pair of boots in the Stoke Bruerne Museum is believed to be puddling boots.

By the 19th century the navvies wore trousers made of moleskin (a thick woollen cloth with a very short pile), double canvas shirts, rainbow coloured waistcoats, velveteen square-tailed coats, gaudy handkerchiefs round their necks and white felt hats. At work they discarded their tail-coats. Although no clothes actually worn by navvies survive, several contemporary prints show navvies dressed in these clothes and contemporary descriptions of them describe the fabrics they were made of and the pride taken in their clothes by the men who made 'the cut', the name given to the canals by those who lived and worked on them.

The later boatmen and their families, however, were better recorded, for the invention and development of photography was contemporary with them and the Stoke Bruerne Museum has many photographs and earlier prints and drawings of the people of the canals. Some of the clothes of the later generations of boat-people survive too, not only at Stoke Bruerne but at Strangers' Hall Museum at Norwich, while there is a boatwoman's bonnet in the industrial history section of Manchester Museum, Manchester University. The few clothes which do survive do not date back before the 1880's and 1890's but the styles worn then had

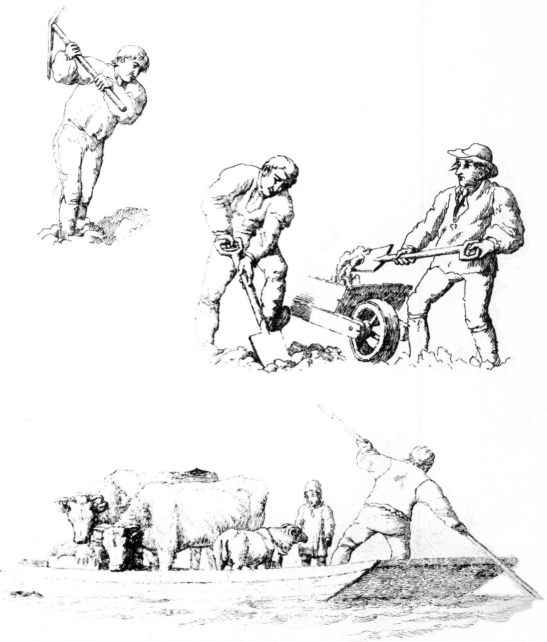

Sketches from W. H. Pyne's *Rustic Figures* 1827

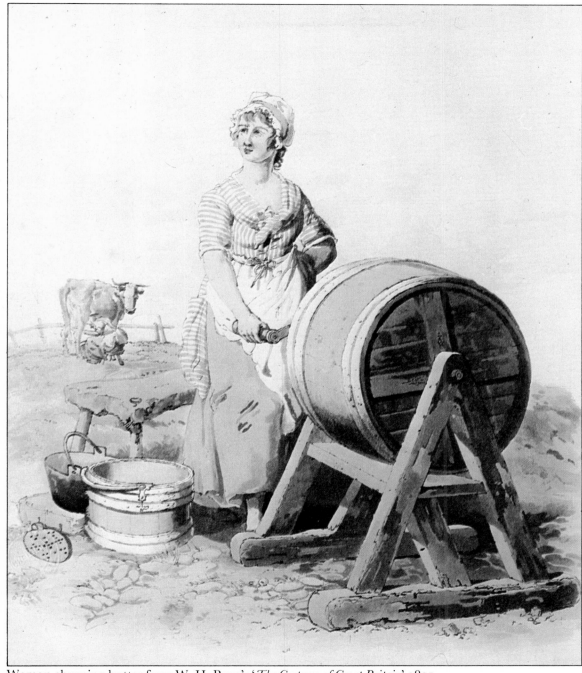

Woman churning butter from W. H. Pyne's '*The Costume of Great Britain*' 1805

become traditional and moved forward into the 20th century, as the 'clothes of the cut'.

To understand how these clothes and the boatmen's way of life evolved we must first study the lives of the canal people before they took to living on the boats. The canals were built as water roads and the first boats to use them were never intended to be family dwellings.

The families of the boatmen lived ashore while the men worked on boats making daily or weekly runs. Most of these boats were owned by Carrying Companies, using double crews and relays of horses to provide a fast carrying service of which they were justifiably proud.

Various theories have been put forward as to the origins of the canal boatmen. It has been suggested that they were gypsies or navvies, or ex-sailors. These theories are open to questioning. Gypsy families would not have lived settled lives in cottages while their menfolk did day or weekly work, and the navvies' characters were often such as would have found regular boatwork dull. The sailors usually came from seaside villages or towns and would have returned there; in addition there is no tradition of nautical terminology on the canals and the biggest insult one could offer to a boatman was to call him 'sailor'. Even their traditional songs mirror this disdain of the sea. However, there is no real proof either for or against these theories. The majority of the boatmen were probably village farm labourers who became unemployed due to the changes in traditional English farming in the late 18th and early 19th centuries. Many of these villagers went to work in the expanding factories of the north and Midlands, but some of them took to boatwork. Although the work was hard, the pay was good (compared with factory workers) and the boatmen were better off than both the factory and the agricultural workers. Boatmen's families often lived on the outskirts of the towns and to some extent had the benefit of the consumer goods made in the towns plus the healthier life of the country.

The people of the late 18th and early 19th centuries have been pictured for us by the pens and brushes of a number of illustrators and painters whose aim was to record the world in which they lived. Among these artists whose work may be seen in museums and art galleries up and down the country are Francis Wheatley, Henri de Cort, George Morland, Thomas Rowlandson, William Hogarth, G. Walker and W. H. Pyne. These last two deliberately set out to depict the working clothes of their fellow-countrymen, and their books and illustrations have been republished since and are an invaluable source of information for social and costume historians. The other artists show people of all classes in their own homes, and from them we learn that although the homes of English working folk were often dark and insanitary and their furniture sparse and simple, they had curtains at their windows, patchwork quilts on their beds, a bird in a cage at the cottage door, crockery on their table and brass jugs and lustre pots on a dresser in their kitchen/living rooms to reflect the firelight at night. The simple cottage furniture of the late 18th and 19th centuries is now valued as antique, as are the china and patchwork of this time, and from the study of them we can learn the tastes of the cottagers, among whom were the boatmen.

The interesting theme that is shown very definitely in all these pictorial records is how slowly the main alterations in fashionable costume affected working people's clothes. Fashionable clothes, worn by upper and middle class women in the early years of the 19th century, were made of flimsy muslin with high waists and wrist-length tight sleeves. Early lithographs and prints, recording the opening of some of the canals show gaily clad passengers of both sexes in open boats pulled by teams of bow haulers. In contrast to the flimsily-dressed middle-class women, the working-class women wear the basic 18th century costume of petticoat and jacket bodice or a petticoat and gown with a bunched-up skirt. With either of these outfits the women wear a large kerchief folded into a triangular scarf around the neck. In most cases their

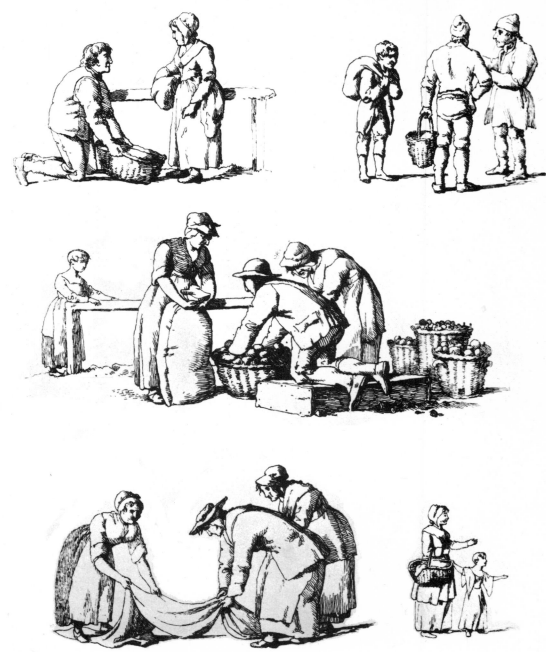

Sketches by W. H. Pyne from 'Rustic Figures' 1827

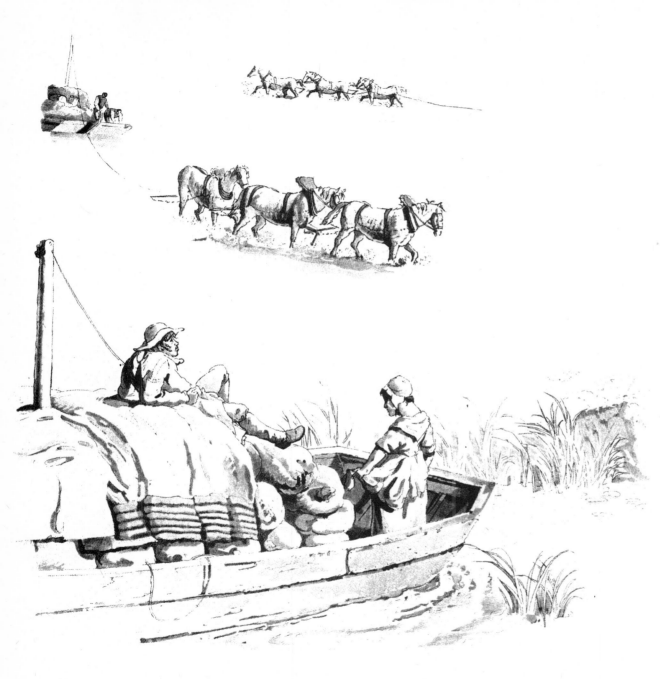

sleeves are wide enough to be rolled up to the elbows or else are made three-quarter length. The boatmen wear boots, breeches, shirts and waistcoats. While the fashionable men wear jackets with tails and fasten their waistcoats below these jackets with studs or buttons, working men wear no jackets and their waistcoats are usually unfastened. W. H. Pyne's drawings show boatmen in very brief waistcoats, looking very like boleros with rolled collars.

In the closing decades of the 18th century only poorer artisans, eccentrics, sailors and small boys wore trousers. The rest wore breeches. W. H. Pyne in 1811 shows inland watermen wearing breeches or trousers. The men loading boats in estuaries or tidal rivers seem to have worn loose trousers, particularly in the eastern counties. Inland, especially in the Midlands, they wore breeches. By the 1840's nearly all men, except those working exclusively with horses as grooms and some farmers (who still wore breeches), wore trousers as a matter of course. These early trousers were cut like sailors' trousers and were fastened with a fall-down flap held by a button each side of the waist. Fly-fronted trousers were introduced in fashionable wear in the 1840's but working men's trousers continued to have front falls until the end of the century.

John Constable painted boats and boatmen in the first three decades of the 19th century. Some of his pictures show boatmen wearing breeches, shirts and waistcoats, but his picture of Flatford Mill painted in 1817, shows a boy on a horse and a man on a boat, both wearing long loose trousers, shirt and waistcoat.

Constable's pictures of canals and boats show men and boys working the boats. Sometimes, as in 'The Leaping Horse', 1825, there are children either on or watching the boats. However, the boats he painted were day boats, many of them the broad barges used in the eastern counties and certainly no boatman's family ever lived on them.

Illustration from W. H. Pyne's '*Microcosm*' 1807

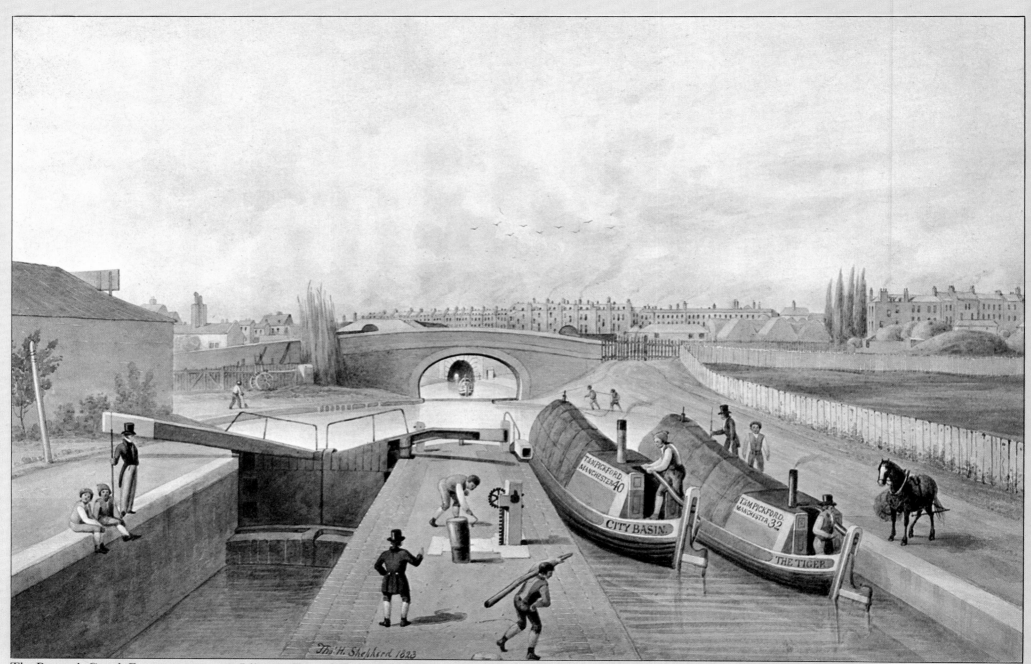

The Regent's Canal, Eastern entrance to Islington Tunnel. Engraved by Thomas Shepherd 1823

2. Competition

Boatwoman's bonnet c. 1880

It was the rising competition of the railways which brought about the beginning of the end of prosperity for the narrow-boatmen and their families. The Carrying Companies cut their men's wages in order to fight back. The usual custom of these companies had been to appoint a boat captain and then leave him to engage another man and a boy as crew. Some captains had bought their boats and often a second and had set up as small carriers. These were known as 'Number Ones' and they were the hardest hit. They could not compete against the faster service of the railways. To save wages in the 1840's whole families left their cottages and moved into the tiny cabins that had never been meant as permanent living quarters; boatmen's wives became the 'second man' and their own small children took the place of 'the boy'. Because these families had known some measure of prosperity the women took their treasured possessions with them to the boats. Into these little cabins they packed the plates, lustre ware, patchwork quilts, brass, fairings and the cage birds that had decorated their cottages. From about this time, too, the narrow boats, which had formerly carried the plain, although bright, colours of the various companies, were decorated with the flowers and castles which have come to be thought of as traditional.

The clothes of these 1840's boatmen, like the clothes of most working men and women, differed from those drawn by Pyne, Morland and Constable. The women no longer wore petticoats with overgowns or jackets. Instead they wore plain waisted dresses with skirts just above the ankle. The white kerchiefs around their shoulders had become small shawls, often of grey or checked wool, while the frilled mob-caps had developed into stiff-brimmed bonnets with a frill hanging down behind. Their menfolk wore corduroy or moleskin trousers, shirts and waistcoats. In winter they wore pea-jackets with high lapels and round billycock hats. Many of the women were skilled needlewomen or lace-makers; their menfolk wore embroidered belts and shirts or fancy braces, their girl children wore print dresses, mob-caps or bonnets like their mothers. The boat decorations, the colours, the deliberate embellishments of ordinary clothes were quite possibly a form of advertising; they had to compete and to do so had first to draw attention to themselves.

Within thirty years the once prosperous boatmen and their families had become some of the poorest and most neglected people in the country. Because they were constantly on the move much of the legislation designed to improve conditions of work and provide education for children could not be applied. Many of the women could not cope with life in the tiny cabins especially with four, five or even more small children. Conditions became insanitary and accidents more common. Many children were drowned each year, many more died of contagious diseases such as typhoid, cholera and smallpox. Although Company boats were supposed to be inspected, it was impossible to enforce the regulations, and in order to get the maximum work out of the boatmen, the Companies tended to turn a blind eye to the conditions of overcrowding which led to ill-temper and frustration, only dispelled by drink with its subsequent ill-treatment of women and children. With speed a necessity, the boatmen had no chance of Sunday rest, no time for church, for education, even for cleanliness or properly cooked food. Everything had to be done 'on the move'. There was no time even for courtship and marriage in the normal way. Marriages were often arranged by mutual acquaintances and contracted for convenience, a young man taking on a boat on his own, asking a friend to find him a woman to travel with. Their 'wedding ceremonies' were arranged by the boaters themselves without the help or blessing of the church. Nobody cared.

It was left to George Smith, a Nonconformist business man of Coalville, Leicester, to campaign on

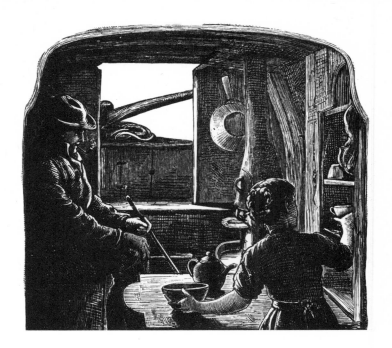

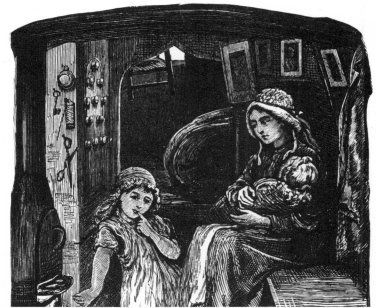

Illustrations of narrow boat cabin from 'The Graphic' 1875

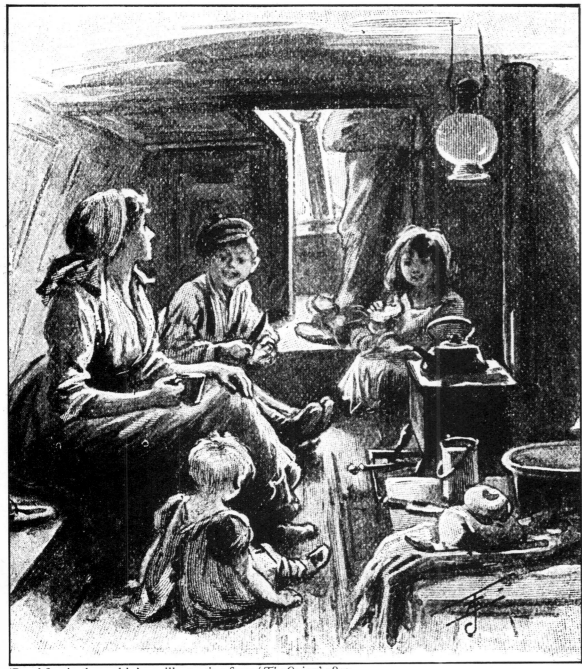

'Breakfast in the cuddy'; an illustration from '*The Quiver*' 1897

the boatpeople's behalf. He had already taken up the cause of the children who worked in brickyards, having himself begun work in a brickyard at the age of nine. By persistence and petitions to Parliament he had obtained an Act to regulate the employment of children in this industry. It was passed in 1872. As a result of this work he lost his own job as manager of a large brickyard and spent the rest of his life in comparative poverty. From 1872 onwards George Smith investigated the conditions of the boats at first-hand, tramping miles of towpath, travelling with the boats and questioning both Canal Company officials and the men, women and children living and working on the boats. He was a tireless writer and petitioner and his books make disturbing reading. Of the 100,000 people he calculated worked on the canals, he estimated that 98% were illiterate and 50% unmarried, all of them living in overcrowded and insanitary conditions. This is a tragic picture of a once gay and independent people. Yet George Smith was a fair investigator and writer. Even as he described the horrors he uncovered he admitted that there were boatmen and women who could cope with life in the cabins and that these were fine and upright people, even if their way of life was different from others. He described the clothes they wore, both good and bad. Of the good he said in 1887 'In walking up Belgrave Gate I came across a real old-fashioned boatwoman, strutting about the streets with a drove of children about her, dressed in her 'Sunday bib and tucker'. She had on a light blue dress, red shawl, with a coal-scuttle kind of green silk velvet bonnet on her head and strong, heavy nailed boots on her feet. She seemed delighted with the fun of showing herself off at Christmastide'. He talks also of 'the sleeved plush-fronted waistcoats, the thick blanket coats and the beloved fur caps, the mighty hob-nailed lace-up boots worn by the boatmen in winter.' But he also speaks of the other side of the picture, of 'the faded woman in rusty ragged attire, half masculine, half feminine, who steered the boat.' Describing a respectable boatman's family, he says he found 'a strong-featured, kindly spoken woman, dressed in the usual reddish-brown nondescript garments, with two little children, a girl of seven and a boy of four, and on her lap, supported by grimy but still all-motherly hands, a tiny, laughing, kicking, crowing month-old boat baby, born in the boat and youngest of five . . . Baby is a great dandy in a nice clean white frock, the whiteness of which . . . contrasts strangely with the dingy surroundings. Somehow, no matter how lowly the parents' lot, the babies always seem to command clean and even gorgeous apparel'. But this was the brighter side of a generally dismal picture.

Thanks to George Smith's efforts and writings, the public's interest in the plight of the boatpeople was aroused. Articles, not only by George Smith, were published in the papers, and these were illustrated by engravings. In the London Illustrated News of October 10th, 1874, a series of plates were published showing aspects of canal boat life. The details of the drawings are not always easy to follow, but they show women in the same plain, ankle-length skirts, shawls and boots that they had first worn on the boats in the 1830's and 1840's. Over the dresses, in some illustrations, they wear a jacket similar to the 18th century 'jacket bodice.'

A reproduction of an engraving of 1875 shows a narrow-boat girl of the Upper Thames, steering a butty. She wears a simple dress with a plain collarless 'Vee' neckline and an apron. The sleeves of the bodice are rolled to just above the elbow and she has a broad plain belt around her waist with a central buckle. It is not possible to tell from this illustration whether the bodice and skirt are separate or not; certainly the bodice is not a jacket bodice and the belt covers the waistband of the apron. Lines over the shoulders of the bodice may mean that she is also wearing a shawl, the ends of which are tucked into the belt at the front. On her head she is wearing a bonnet with a plain stiffened front brim, the crown gathered into this, while a long frill known as a curtain can be seen blowing across from the back of the bonnet. The significant fact about this bonnet is that it has no

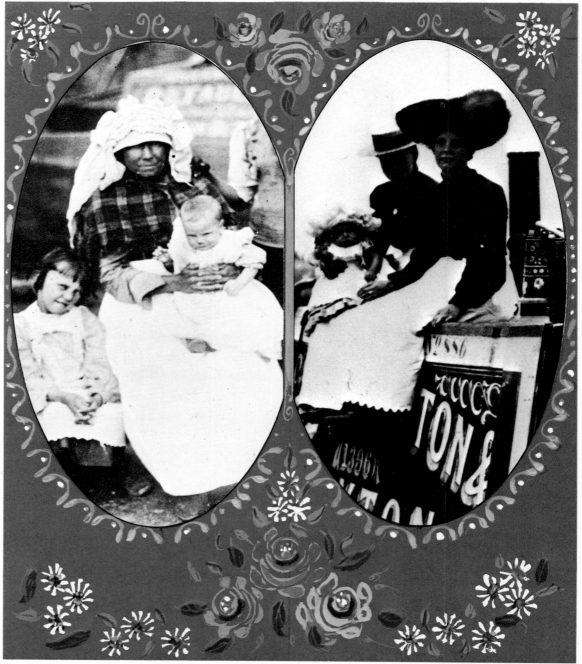

Canal babies, early 1900's

16

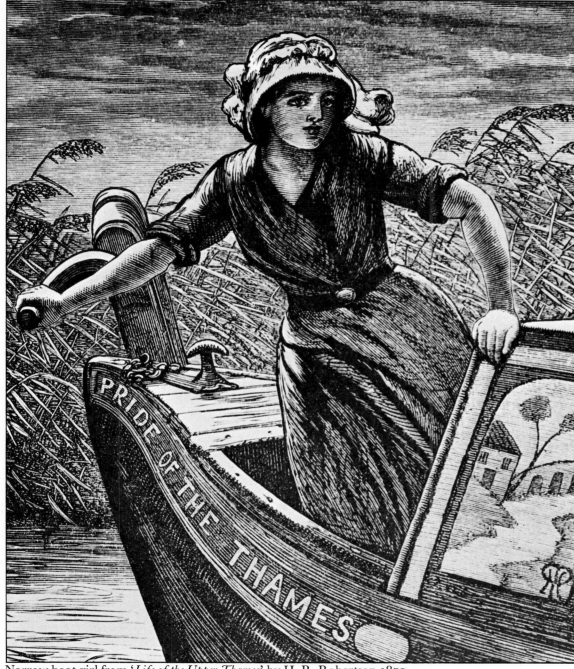

Narrow boat girl from '*Life of the Upper Thames*' by H. R. Robertson 1875

strings and is more like a hat pulled well down on the head. If it has strings they are mixed into the folds of the curtain and are blown back from the girl's head. The whole picture betokens a windy day.

The men in the engravings of the 1870's wear fairly wide trousers, shirts and waistcoats, with high lapelled, straight-cut jackets over the top in winter. In the illustration 'Tea-time on a Monkey Boat' the man outside the cabin wears a 'billycock hat', while the man inside wears a soft cap with ear-flaps turned up. The general atmosphere of this picture indicates fog and bad weather.

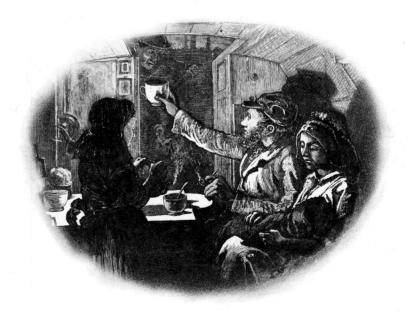

Canal life '*Teatime on a Monkey Boat*' Illustrated London News 1874

17

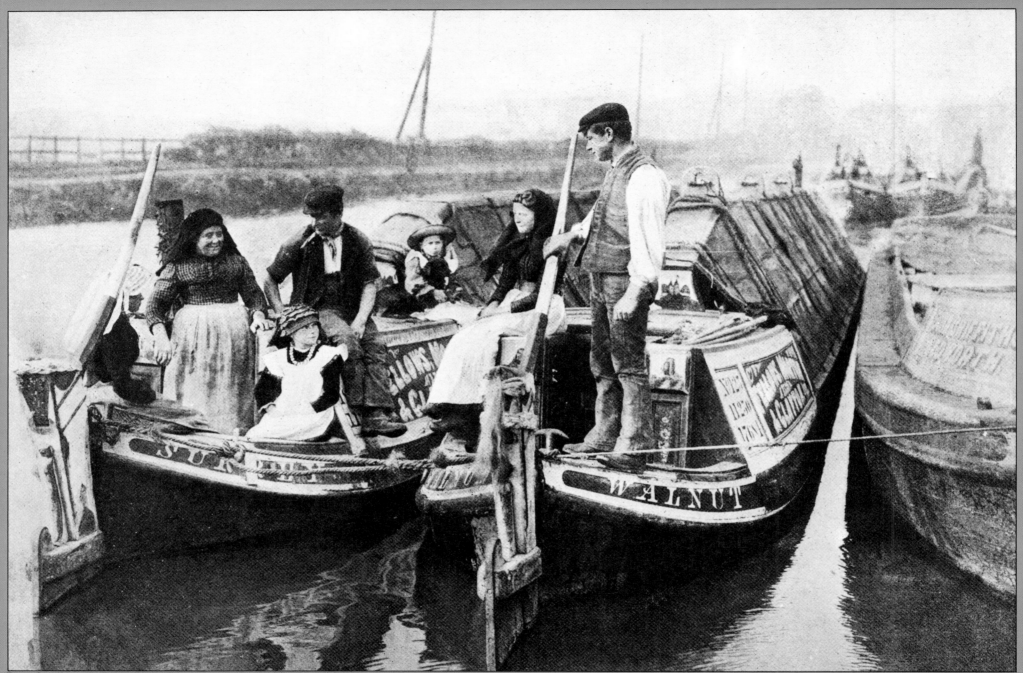

Boat family near Brentford – Photograph from '*The Graphic*' 1910

3. Flowering of a Tradition

Boatwoman and boatman c. 1900

In 1877, largely as a result of the work of George Smith, the Canal Boats Act was passed. It was a start in the betterment of the boatmen's lives, but it did not satisfy George Smith because it was too permissive and could not be enforced. The children continued to live on the boats and remained uneducated. He went on campaigning and an amendment to the Act was passed in 1881. In 1884 a second Canal Boats Act was passed, appointing an inspector under the Local Government Board. It also required local authorities to make annual reports to this Board concerning actions they had taken over supervising canal life and to see that boat children attended schools. Slowly, very slowly, the boatpeople's lives improved; though many children remained unlettered, general conditions and hours of work were easier. As conditions of health improved so the boaters' pride returned; the decorated boats and clothes took on a new meaning to their owners. The 'traditional' way of life, the best of the canal songs and dances, the brightest costumes date from the 1890's onward, and it is these clothes and domestic utensils which are preserved as the tradition of the cut.

Even the Canal Companies caught something of this new spirit. Some of them supplied clothes to their employees. The captains and mates of Fellows, Morton and Clayton's steam-driven narrow boats between 1880 and 1920 were given corduroy trousers, wide leather belts, brass-buttoned waistcoats with velvet collars, striped shirts, coloured neckerchiefs and braided braces. They had jackets, too, also with velvet collars, and flat caps. While the jackets, judging by the photographs of these men, were often discarded, the caps were worn even on the hottest days. Lock keepers were also given distinguishing clothes to wear. The Peak Forest Canal Minute Books record that their lock keepers and toll keepers were to be provided

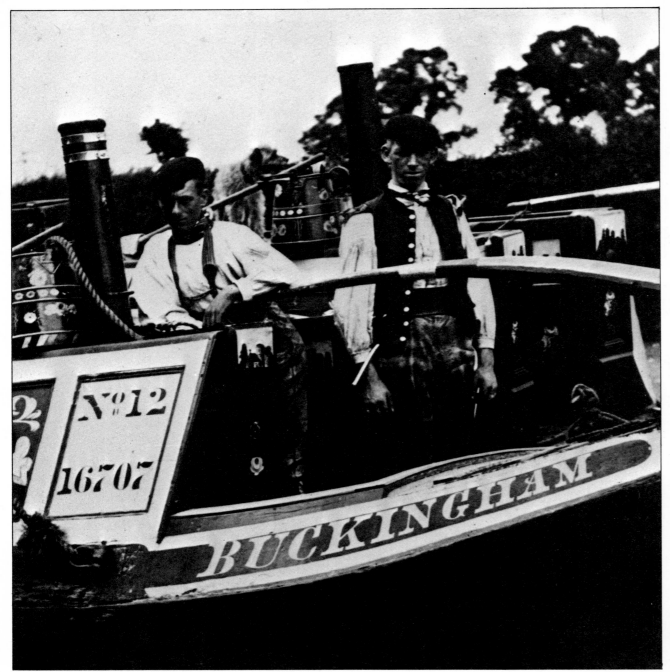

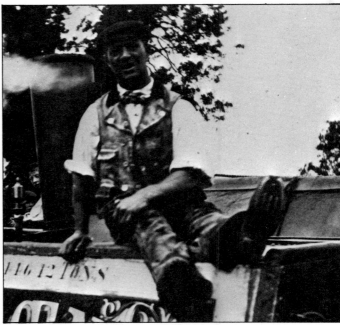

Fellows, Morton & Clayton uniform c. 1910

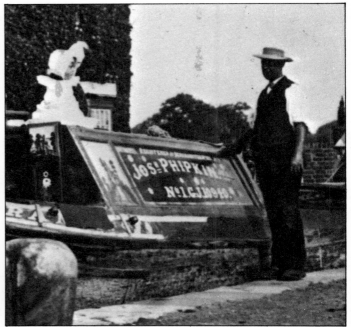

Fellows, Morton & Clayton uniform (between 1880 and 1920)

Joseph Phipkin and baby at Buckby Locks c. 1912

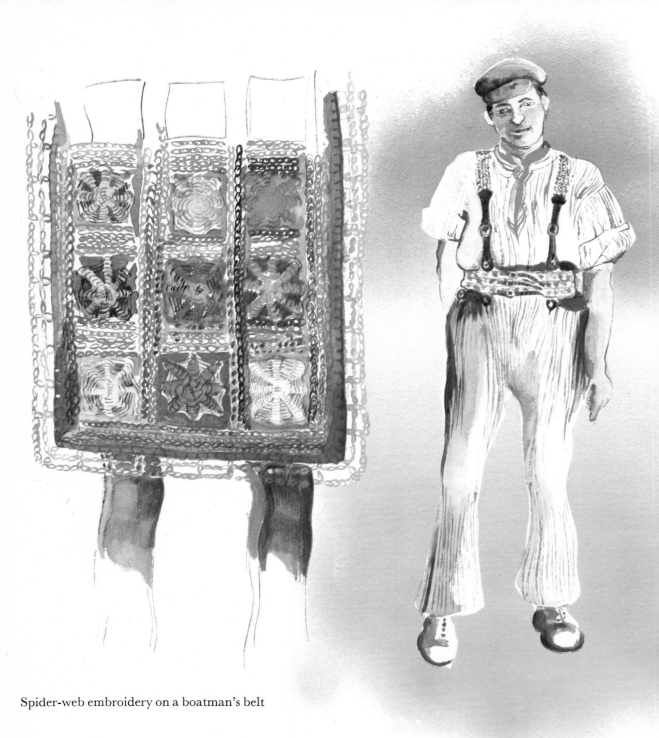

with 'an upper waistcoat and a badge thereon to distinguish them from other persons.'

The 'Number Ones', the boatmen owning their own boats, wore similar clothes to those issued by the Companies and were proud of being different from people 'off the land.' Corduroy or moleskin trousers were worn with striped shirts, neckerchiefs and waistcoats. Their boats were decorated with painted flowers and castles; the cabins inside were further decorated with lace plates and crochet curtains. Their clothes were also decorated with embroidery. A man's shirt on show in the Stoke Bruerne Museum is embroidered in red feather-stitching down the front. The shirts worn were collarless and a handkerchief or scarf was folded round the neck-band instead of the stiff collars worn by men of indoor occupations. By the 1890's boatmen were able to buy suits, trousers with matching jackets and waistcoats. Usually they wore black flared trousers, cut with front falls at the waist, a waistcoat with a 'keyhole' shaped neckline, showing off the embroidered shirt above it, and a high lapelled jacket. Even for best, the boatman wore his coloured neckerchief, rather than a collar. The outfit was completed with the flat cap or trilby hat and black boots. Another typical suit was made in a small check material of black and brown, the trousers again being cut with front falls. Boatmen made their own fashions and probably found the old-fashioned cut of trousers more comfortable. Their waistcoats were cut straight at the waist while fashionable waistcoats were cut with points.

At work, as the photographs in the Stoke Bruerne Museum show, they did not wear suit jackets; if it was very cold they still wore the short thick coats that have been variously known since about 1800 as pea-jackets, monkey-jackets or reefers. They were similar in cut to a modern duffle coat, although slightly shorter.

The men still wore their waistcoats undone, showing their shirts; often they wore both belt and braces. One of the belts in the Stoke Bruerne collection is of leather, decorated with brass studs, others are made of stout

Spider-web embroidery on a boatman's belt

canvas covered with embroidery that resembles a spider-web pattern of many colours. The origin of this emboidery is unknown; the 'webs' are set in squares about one inch in size and the stitches resemble the spokes of a wheel. The pattern is not found in any other form of traditional English embroidery, such as the 19th century countrymen's smocks, nor is it a stitch used in the heavily embroidered baby gowns of the 19th century. Like the painted flowers and castles on the boats, it seems to belong to 'the cut'. Braces too were ornamented and coloured, often made of complicated plaits of multi-coloured wools. Again, the origins of these are obscure, as they seem only to have been worn by boatmen, but it is possible that the patterns date from the days before the families lived on the boats. Some of the wives of boatmen may have been straw-plaiters in the 1830's, as the pattern of the plaiting parallels some of the patterns used for plaits for straw hat making. This skill may have been passed on and used in making the braces, which were made by the boatwomen for their menfolk. In the Stoke Bruerne Museum there is a matching plaited belt and braces set in red, black and yellow wool.

The clothes worn by the women were no less distinctive and different from the clothes of women 'off the land'. By the late 1880's and 1890's they consisted of an ankle length skirt, a blouse, sometimes worn tucked inside the skirt, often worn outside, a long apron, a shawl and a bonnet. The skirts, to judge by the photographs of boatwomen, were commonly striped and decorated with bands round the hem. Of the boatwomen's skirts which survive, the one in Norwich Museum is of navy drill, with narrow red and white stripes. This is banded with the same material, cut on the cross. The boatwoman's 'best' skirt, in Stoke Bruerne Museum, is made of pink and white striped material banded at the hem with three black ribbon bands. A child's skirt in the same museum is black, with added stripes of pink, green, red and yellow giving an embroidered effect.

The blouses worn by boatwomen were influenced slightly by land fashions, in as much as many of the

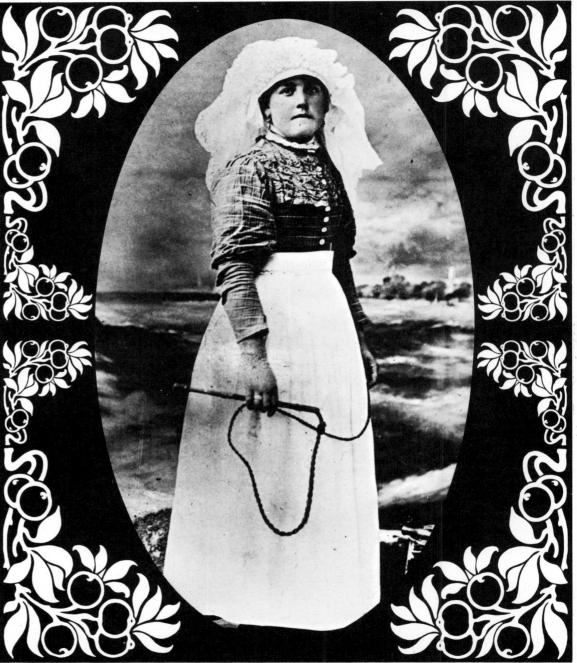

Boatwoman c. 1904

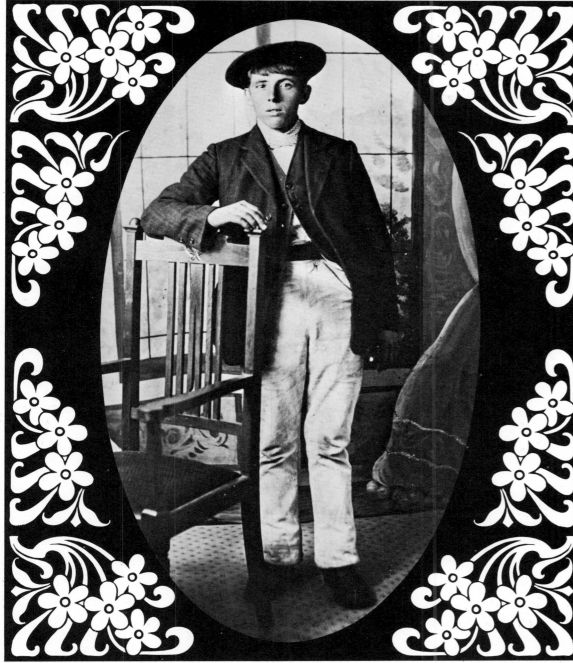

Boatman c. 1900

photographs show leg-of-mutton sleeves and tucked bodices being worn. The surviving blouses also show these features. They were made in a variety of patterns, fabrics and colours, black or grey being popular among older women; striped winceyette, similar to men's shirting, or small flower-sprigged cottons were popular among younger women. White does not appear to have been worn for blouses, and among surviving clothes of any sort there are none made in the reddish-brown colour that George Smith seems to have found so commonly worn.

White was reserved for aprons and bonnets, although to judge by the photographs a fawn holland (often used for making working women's aprons) seems to have been worn as well. However, the white aprons predominate. These aprons were large, covering the whole of the front of the skirt. They were gathered into waistbands and had no bibs. In cold weather a shawl was worn about the boatwoman's shoulders, pinned in front so that she could use her hands freely. When made of woven fabrics they were usually a grey, black, and white plaid, but many photographs show women in crocheted shawls and both a plaid shawl and a pink crocheted shawl are in the Stoke Bruerne collection.

The most popular craft among the boatwomen was crochet and their best clothes were lavishly edged with crochet lace. It was used on aprons, blouse frills and bonnets. In the cabins crocheted lace curtains were draped around the bed place and even the boathorse was given a crocheted ear-protector to keep away the flies. In the Stoke Bruerne Museum are two such ear-protectors decorated with coloured tassels. Some boatwomen kept a cage-bird which travelled on the cabin top in fine weather and this, too, would have a crocheted cage cover. Crochet work could be done while travelling and kept in a pocket when both hands were on the tiller or full attention needed at locks. The boatwomen were very proud of this crochet work and would probably compete with each other in its use as decoration.

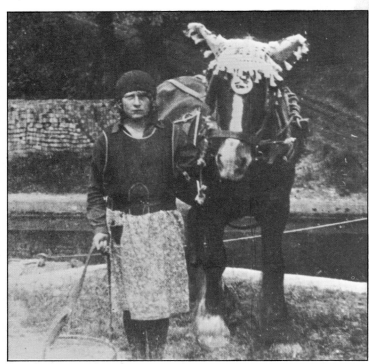

Boat horse wearing ear protector, c. 1930

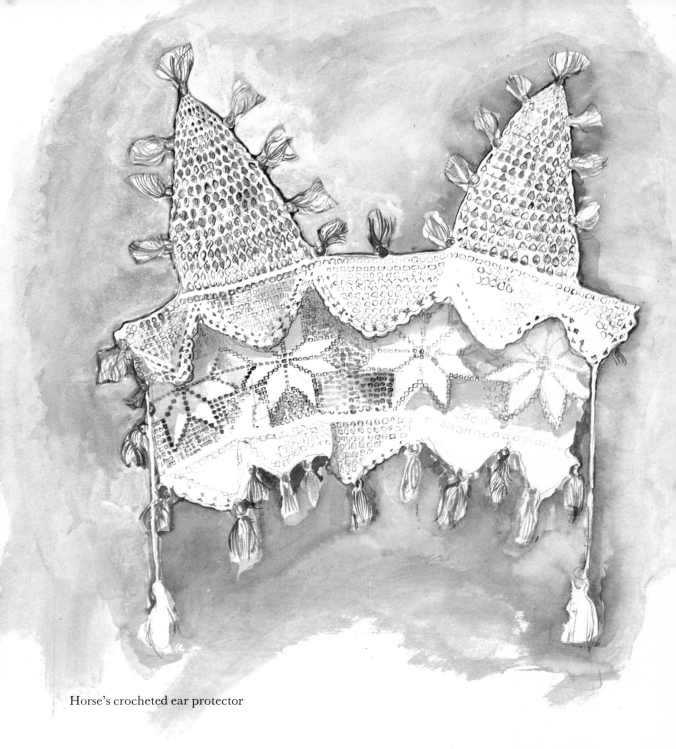

Horse's crocheted ear protector

24

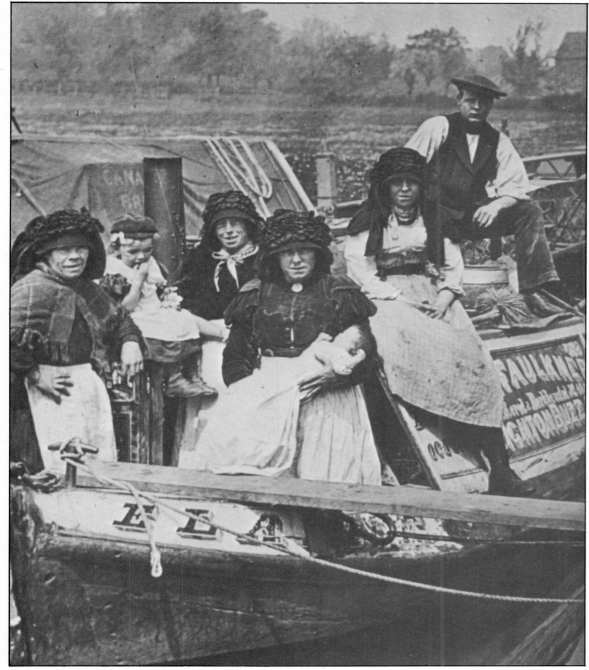

Christening Party 1913.

But the real distinguishing feature of a boatwoman's costume was her bonnet. During the 19th century women had gradually abandoned the mob cap and straw hat of the early decade in favour of a bonnet with a stiffened brim across the front and a frill, known as a 'curtain', hanging over the shoulders. The design of these bonnets (which were worn by practically all labouring classes of English women, especially those who spent long hours out of doors) varied from region to region. Those worn by fruit-pickers in Kent were the simplest in design. The more complicated designs were worn by the women of the Midlands and the most elaborate of these by the boatwomen. The stiff brims were formed by rows of corded quilting, the main part of the bonnet by alternate rows of frilled tucks and gathered cording. A horse-shoe shaped piece of corded and quilted fabric at the back shaped it to the head, while the curtain was much longer than general, often double, and in the more embellished bonnets, edged with crochet lace and decorated with bows and streamers of the fabric. Although made with strings that could be tied under the chin, these were often left undone to hang down in front. The bonnet was, in reality, a bonnet-shaped hat, being extremely practical as well as decorative. It effectively kept off both rain and sun and could be tied firmly in place in windy weather.

In the 1880's and 90's these bonnets were made of white or small flower-sprigged cotton. In 1901 when Queen Victoria died the nation plunged into almost universal mourning; even the poorest boatwoman made herself a black bonnet, the same pattern as the white or flower-sprigged bonnet of the previous decade, and these continued thereafter to be worn until the 1920's and 30's. A photograph in the Stoke Bruerne Museum shows a christening party of 1913 on board a narrow boat and all four women in the picture are wearing elaborate black bonnets. So universal were these black bonnets that L. T. C. Rolt, in his book *Narrow Boat* written in the late 1930's, describes the black bonnet as the traditional wear of the boatwomen. The black bonnet was lined with

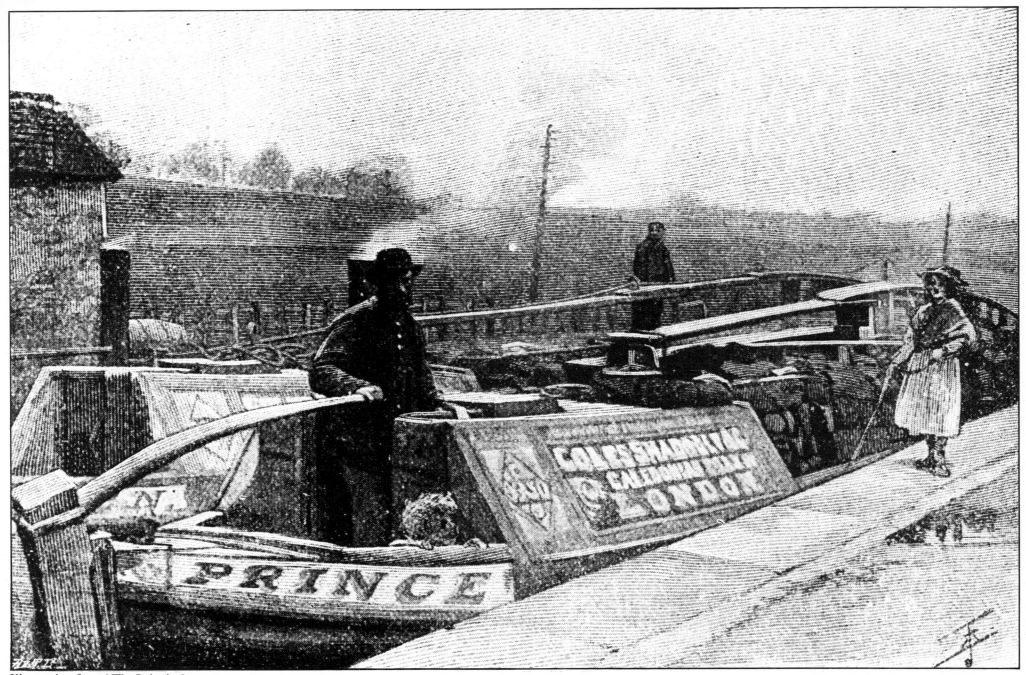

Illustration from '*The Quiver*' 1897

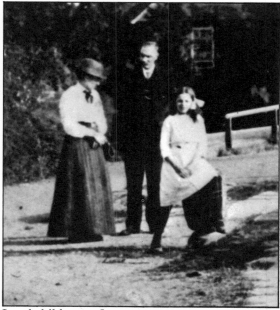

Land child c. 1906

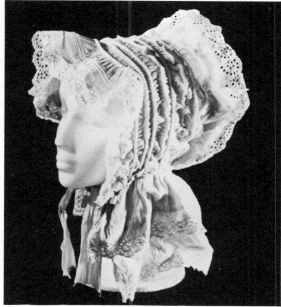

Boat baby's bonnet 1903–1912

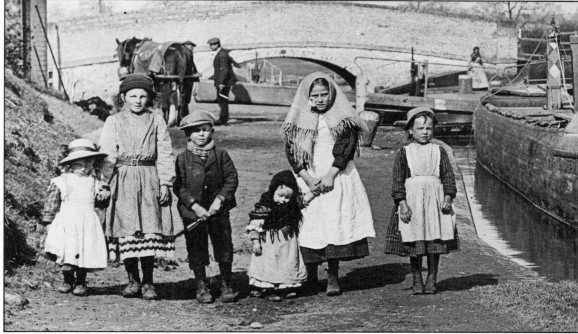

Edward Powell's children at Braunston Top Lock c. 1914

waterproof material and could therefore have been worn in both summer and winter.

From 1914 some boatwomen, noticeably the younger women, took to wearing some fashionable clothes, including large hats. These hats, though, were the high fashion wear of the years 1906–1910. Being large they probably provided more protection than the fashionable little cloches of the war years. A young boatwoman photographed wearing a straw boater probably considered herself as fashionable as any girl 'off the land'. Hats seem to have been worn for weddings and funerals too, although, a few years before, all the women would have worn bonnets.

The boat children, for whose sakes George Smith campaigned so vigorously, appear in the photographs taken in the 1890's to be happy and plump. They may not have had much schooling, for even after the passing of the 1884 Act many remained illiterate, but they appear adequately clothed and well cared for. It was not until 1920 that a Boat Children's Education Act was passed which specified that such children must attend school for at least 200 days a year. Schools were opened in boats at the main canal centres and children attended them during loading and unloading times. Others became weekly or short term boarders at such schools. In the 1940's one Midlands Local Authority opened a boarding school for boat children who returned to their parents' floating homes during the holidays.

All this has come to pass in the lifetime of the small children who appear in the 1890's and 1900's photographs at Stoke Bruerne. As babies they are gorgeously dressed in the lavishly embroidered robes common to all artisan babies of the times. As toddlers they wear older children's cast-offs, even the boys wearing, for a few years at least, dresses and pinafores like their sisters. Often they are also swathed in large scarves, firmly pinned behind. The girls wear bonnets that are more simply made than their mothers', being just a white cap with a frill. These children's bonnets are also worn by older girls and young women. Boys

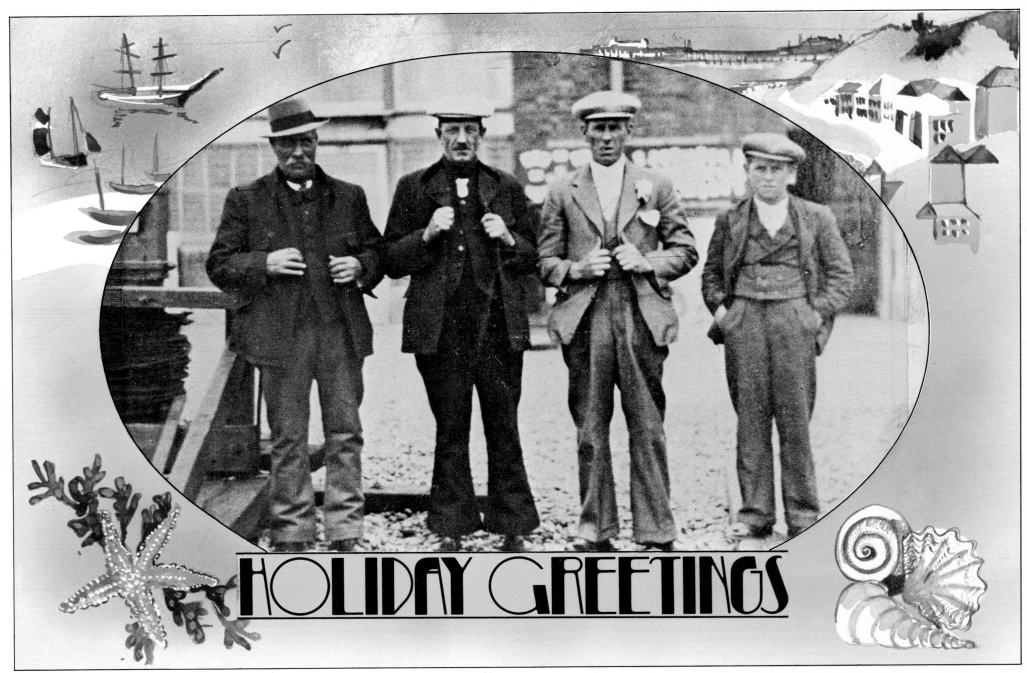

Number Ones on holiday at Brighton in the early 1930's

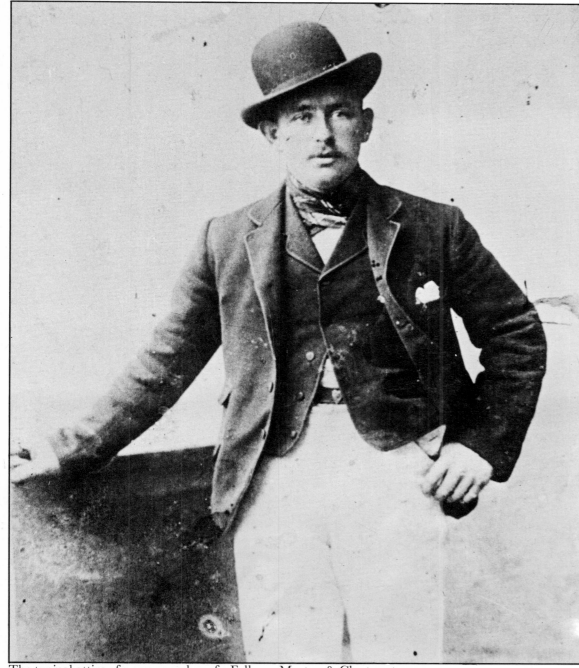

The typical attire of a crewmember of a Fellows, Morton & Clayton steamer

seem to have worn flat caps like their fathers from the age of five. The 1890's photographs show small boys wearing short trousers to just below the knee; with these short trousers they wear shirts and incongruously adult-looking waistcoats. Only in the photographs dating from the 1920's do we see the beginning of the end of the traditional costume—boys and girls in knitted jerseys, the girls in short knee-length skirts wearing berets instead of the traditional bonnets. Even in the 1920's however, the women and girls continued to wear the high, laced boots that had always been worn by the boatwomen; prior to this they had been hidden by the longer skirts.

Men's clothes, too, were beginning to change. From the turn of the century the Number Ones had begun to wear bowler hats. By the 1920's these hard hats were as common as the flat caps of the 1880's and 1890's. A cap survives at Stoke Bruerne, but the bowlers can only be seen in the photographs.

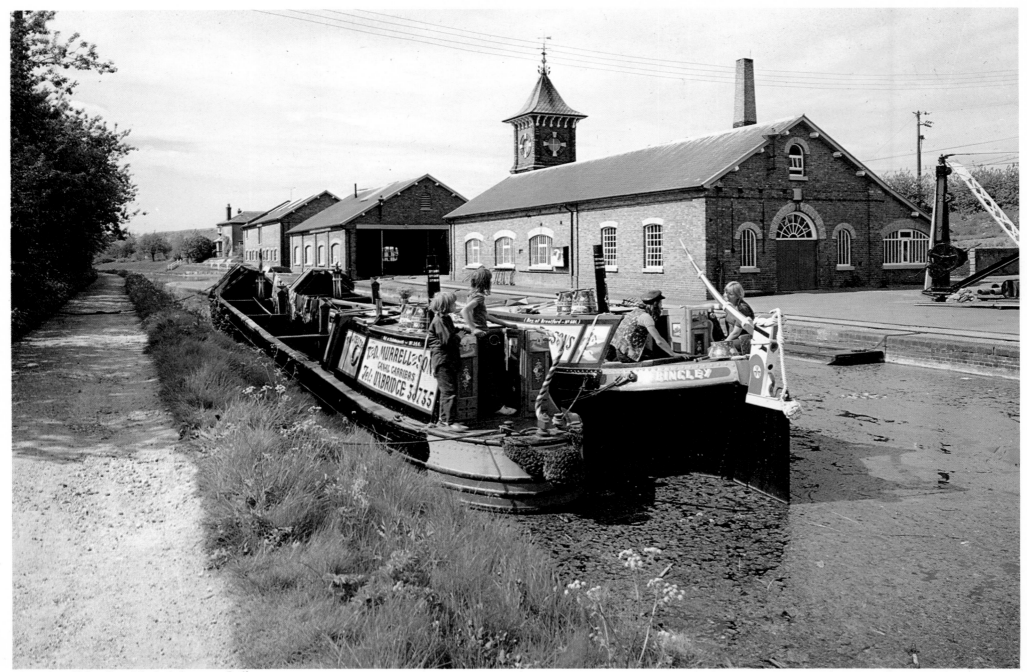

The Murrell family with their boats at Bulbourne 1974

The traditional narrow-boat clothes are no longer worn; there are very few working boats now and their captains wear modern jeans if they are young, and flannels and old jackets if they are middle aged. In the summer the young men wear their jeans without a shirt, a practice that would have horrified the boatmen of the 18th and 19th centuries. Although a few of the older boatmen still live in retirement on boats neither they nor their wives wear the traditional clothes of the cut. To find these now one must go to the Waterways Museum at Stoke Bruerne, where not only the clothes of the boatpeople are displayed but photographs, prints, documents, parts of boats and all the other items which made up the daily life of the boatmen can be seen. It is hoped that this booklet will lead to a greater understanding of both the difficulties and the differences between the lives of those of us 'off the land' and the people of 'the cut'.

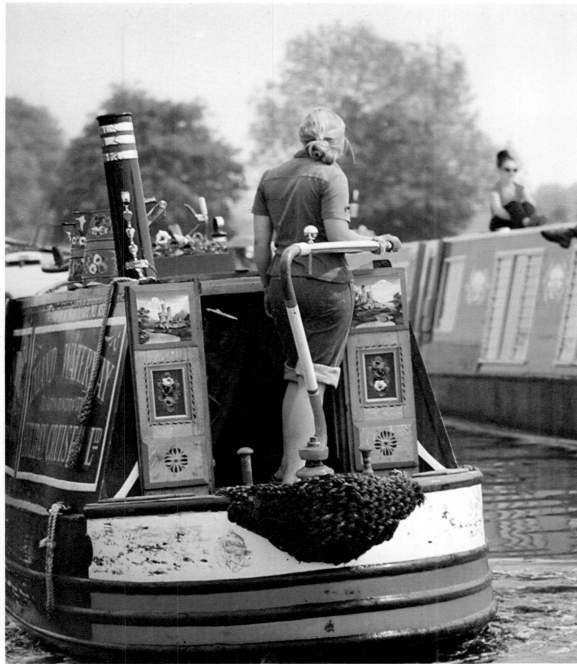

Hotel boats on the Shropshire Union Canal 1975

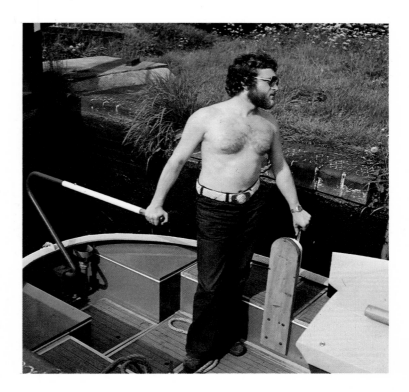

Appendix
A GENERAL INTRODUCTION TO COUNTRY AND WORKING CLOTHES OF THE 19th CENTURY

One of the difficulties of research into working clothes of past centuries is that so few of them survive. There are many fashionable clothes in museums up and down the country, but taken alone they give a wrong impression of life in the past. In the past fashion moved down the social scale very slowly, in spite of the fact that all through the 18th and 19th centuries fashion writers were constantly bewailing that the poorer people 'aped their betters'. In many cases they just could not afford to, or the fashionable clothes were unsuitable for work.

An important factor that influenced workpeoples' taste was the enormous trade in second-hand clothes. Among the 'lower orders', a best dress may well have had several owners so that there was an enormous time lag in fashions among the different classes and country women's clothes could be anything up to thirty years out of date according to fashionable circles. All this makes for social distinction and in the 19th century paintings and writings the different social classes can easily be distinguished by their clothes. The working, and working class, clothes of the early 19th century had their origins in the fashionable clothes of the 18th century. The exception is the change over from breeches to trousers, by men in the early years of the 19th century, a true case of 'fashion in reverse' in which the upper classes adopted the clothes of the very lowest.

In general terms, people of all classes but especially the fashionable, tended to wear more and more clothes as the century went on. This is particularly noticeable in children's clothes; the babies, in Regency times, wore a quarter or less of the weight of clothes worn by babies in the 1890's. Adult underclothes and the fabrics other clothes were made from also gradually became heavier as the century progressed. With the added weight came an added sense of propriety and some of the old terms for clothes were deemed improper and new euphemisms devised. This occasionally makes research into literary sources comical, for the names of clothes may come to mean quite different garments to later generations. In the following notes I have used the modern terms, explaining the earlier ones where necessary.

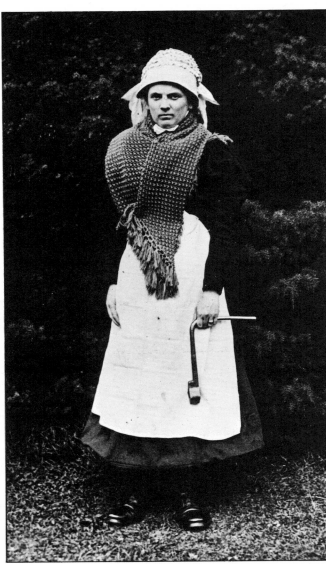

Narrow boatwoman on the River Nene 1897

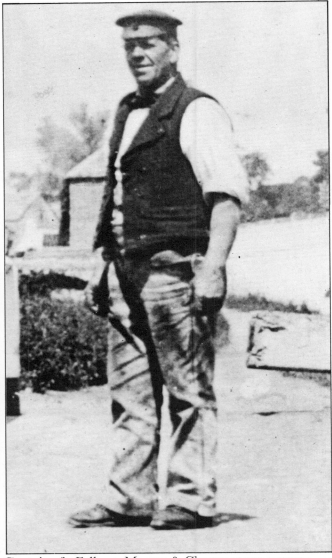

Captain of a Fellows, Morton & Clayton steam narrow boat 1897

Women

Underclothes

For centuries women's normal undergarment was a straight, short-sleeved linen garment. This was called a 'shift' up to the end of the 18th century and became known as a 'chemise' in the 19th century. Its length could be anything between knee and ankle and at various times in the past, drawers have been worn beneath it or not, according to the fashion of the time and the social class of the wearer. Over this was worn the corset, called 'stays' in the 18th century. This was not necessarily an undergarment and the working dress of the country women was often just a shift, stays, 'petticoat' and neckerchief, put on in that order. The shift is the garment that looks like a short-sleeved blouse in 18th century paintings of country girls. A 'petticoat' was simply a skirt, gathered to a waistband; a woman could wear as many as three on top of each other, each a little shorter than the one below, so that different bands of colour showed at the hem. Only in the 19th century was it considered indecent to show the shift and a 'petticoat' became an underskirt that was not visible. But this, and the change of nomenclature, was only a fashionable innovation; paintings of country girls in the 1860's and 1870's still show them wearing versions of the petticoat and stays with a neckerchief as their great-grandmothers wore in the 18th century.

Skirts

Many poorer working class women wore plain gathered skirts (the top 'petticoat') all through the century. They were usually made of two widths of material at the beginning of the century and grew wider (three widths) in the 1850's and 1860's. When fashionable women wore crinolines, working class women's skirts looked skimpy; when fashionable women wore narrower skirts at the end of the century, working women's skirts seemed full. In fact they had not changed except to revert to the two widths of material in the 1890's. Country girls often decorated their skirts by sewing contrasting bands in rows above the hem – this was only very occasionally a fashionable decoration (c. 1850's and during the 1870's) being a 'peasant' type of decoration, common to all of Europe, although only a very poor version of it was ever used in England. Bustles were worn by village girls in the 1880's and these persisted into the 1890's, but were no more than a pad or pillow pinned beneath the skirt.

Bodices

Over their stays, country women and working girls wore jacket bodices. This 'jacket and petticoat' has been more or less a basic working woman's dress since the 16th century, although all fashionable dress has influenced it to some extent, especially in the cut of the neckline and the sleeve. All women want to be fashionable, no matter how poor, and there is none of the traditional peasant 'national costume' in England, engendering local pride. The most that can be said of the 19th century working women's costume was that it was as plain as possible, until towards the end of the century when most women had a 'best dress' or bodice which was as near the fashion as they could get. The linen kerchiefs of the 18th century became in the 19th century the small shawls worn over the shoulders, especially in the North and Midlands. These were sometimes knitted or crocheted, but more often a grey, white and black plaid.

By the 1880's, when cheap printed cotton was available, most women had a bodice, sometimes a skirt as well, in this fabric. The patterns were small, printed in pink, blue, green and lilac, on white, often in tiny stripes of flowers. Usually the bodice was patterned and the skirt made of a plain, darker material. Striped fabric (woven, not printed) was sometimes used for working class dresses, and by the end of the century a heavy checked calico was used for summer skirts. After 1901 (Queen Victoria's death) many working class women went into black clothes, and continued to wear them until the 1920's.

One-piece Dresses – Gowns

In the 18th century a 'gown' was a one-piece dress. It could be an 'open-fronted' gown, with its skirt open to show the petticoat or it could be a 'round gown' with no front opening. Among working women it was a 'best' dress (if they had one) and would not be worn while actually working. It was invariably behind the times as far as the fashionable world was concerned. A 'bedgown' in 18th century terms was simply an informal dress (it was certainly never worn in bed). Basically a 'bedgown' was a one-piece waisted dress with its skirt and its bodice open to the waist. It was worn over petticoat and stays, and we would think of it as a 'coat dress'. Fashionable women wore 'bedgowns' in the 18th century as an informal morning costume; working women looked on it as everyday wear and its skirt could be any length from thigh to ankle. When short, it became the 'jacket bodice' already mentioned. When long, its skirts were bunched up behind to give a bustle effect and get the loose sides of the open front out of the way, in which case it still looked a little like a jacket. By the 1840's the 'round gowns', formerly only worn for best, had become more general wear, especially among younger working women, and the 'bedgown' had lost its name and finally become a proper, skirted jacket, often worn over a 'gown'. From the 1860's onward, best dresses were often two-piece, meeting or fastening together at the waist. The time lag in fashion gets shorter as the 19th century went by. The thirty year fashion gap of the beginning of the century narrowed to between five and ten years by the end, except in communities that had either little contact with the fashionable world, such as the Yorkshire Dales, or, like the boat people, attempted to preserve an identity in spite of dispersion.

Bonnets

Country girls wore white caps under straw or stiff bonnets at the beginning of the century. By the 1860's the caps, except for older women, were abandoned, and country girls wore sunbonnets. These tended to vary in their patterns, those of the Midlands (and subsequently those of boatwomen) being more elaborate than those of Berkshire or Surrey. Those worn in Kent were plainest of all. Basically a sunbonnet is a cap with a forward projecting brim and a curtain to shade the neck. The elaboration consists of the numbers of rows of frills, cording and quilting across the top and brim, and the numbers of layers of 'curtains' at the back. From 1870 to 1901 these were made in sprigged cotton. In 1901 many were made in black cotton (especially in the Midlands and the North). Children, young girls and babies wore white sunbonnets without the very elaborate curtains, just a single frill at the back.

Aprons.

These were worn over the petticoats and jackets, or 'bedgowns'. Long, bibless aprons of white or brown linen (or later holland) were usually worn. By the end of the century some aprons had bibs back and front, with wide shoulder straps edged with broad frills. When these were worn over a petticoat and shift, it gave the effect of a modern 'pinafore dress'. Although worn by many working women this type of pinafore does not seem to have been worn by boatwomen.

Illustrations from W. H. Pyne's '*The Costume of Great Britain*' 1805

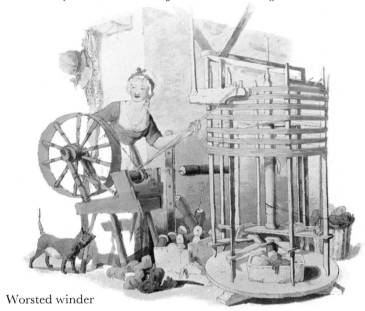

Worsted winder

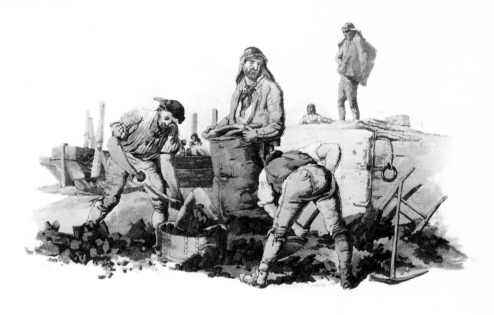

Coal heavers

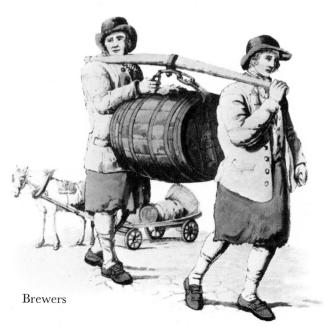

Brewers

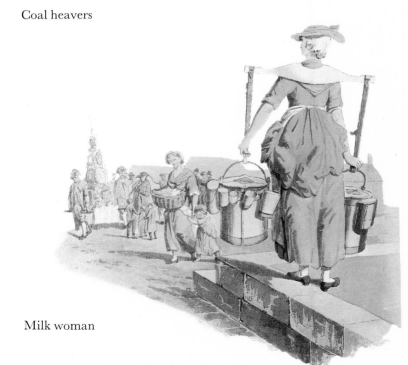

Milk woman

Men

Trousers

During the 18th century all men wore breeches. They were commonly known as 'small clothes'. The front opening was in the form of a flap, known as a 'fall down' front or 'spair'. In the unfashionable or working men's trousers this extended across the whole front and was called 'whole falls' while fashionable breeches had a flap ranging from 5 in.–9in. wide and called 'small' or 'split' falls. Behind the fall down flap a band reached from side to side and was buttoned at the centre. This band, known as the 'bearer' was some 5 in. deep in the middle and 7 in. or 8 in. at the sides; it rose a couple of inches above the top of the fall. When this band was narrow it was called a 'French bearer' but when very deep a 'Bilston' bearer. The latter was commonly worn by the elderly and the manual labouring class.

Trousers were first worn at Brighton by fashionable young men in 1807, but by 1830 had replaced breeches entirely for fashionable wear, except for ceremonial or court occasions. Countrymen continued to wear breeches, but labourers and town manual workers wore trousers with their front openings made as a flap, like the breeches. Fly fronts were first used in fashionable trousers in the 1820's but were still thought indelicate even by 1830. Fly fronts became fashionable in the 1840's, but unfashionable trousers continued to be made with front falls almost until the end of the century.

Fashionable trousers were unlined, but among the working classes and small tradesmen the 'Sunday best' trousers, usually of black broadcloth, were lined with either coarse white canvas or thick twilled cotton, and such specimens from the second half of the 19th century may still be found. Corduroy trousers originated with the 'navvies' who dug the canals and built the railways. These men wore trousers (as did small boys) before the Prince Regent set the fashion for them at Brighton, and long before other labouring men wore trousers. These corduroy trousers were passed down from one generation to another, being apparently incapable of being worn out, but they can sometimes be dated by their buttons, although it must be remembered that buttons are often replaced. Trouser buttons of bone or brass with two holes are pre-1830, between 1830–1840 these had four holes, while after 1840 buttons were made of black japanned iron with four holes.

The legs of fashionable trousers have been cut in various widths since 1807, but navvies' trousers and labouring trousers were usually 'full gaitered bottomed' i.e. cut with a slight flare. A string, called a 'york' or a 'lijah' in the eastern counties was often tied round just below the knee.

Waistcoats

Labouring classes did not follow fashion, and 19th century waistcoats for working men followed the late 18th century with high stand-up collars. They were often worn instead of jackets, to show the sleeves of the shirt, which were usually rolled up, especially in the case of the navvies. These waistcoats were seldom buttoned. Sleeved waistcoats were worn by ostlers and by mid-century by railway porters. These were always buttoned up as they were regarded as part of a livery or uniform. Some boatmen seem to have worn sleeved waistcoats in the 1850's and 1860's. The metal buttons often have the maker's name and a date stamped on them; sometimes these buttons were detachable, the shanks passing through eyeletted holes and held at the back with split pins.

Shirts

18th century and early 19th century shirts were cut very wide, shorter than worn today, with no tails. They were collarless, the neck being gathered into a band, and the sleeves gathered into a very low shoulder seam. These shirts did not open right down the front (the coat shirt is a post-1945 product of the 20th century) and early shirts were sometimes fastened by laces, not buttons. Shirts got narrower as the 19th century progressed and colours were introduced generally in labourers' shirts in the second half of the century, in the form of narrow stripes or cross stripes. Early shirts made of linen, later of twilled cotton or 'wincyette'; side slits and tails were introduced as shirts became narrower.

Underclothes

During the 18th and early 19th century labouring men did not wear underclothes. The shirt itself was considered an undergarment and was very seldom seen without a waistcoat on top of it. An extra shirt, or an overall cut like a shirt could be worn instead of a jacket, and eventually became the countryman's smock; although made in a thicker material than the linen used for shirts, it was cut to the same basic pattern as the 18th century shirt.

Vests and underpants came in in the mid 19th century for labouring men and at first were probably worn only by the elderly. The working class trousers were lined with cotton or twill and only the fashionable and middle class wore separate underpants. But as the 19th century passed more and more clothes were worn. The Victorians were responsible for the theory that 'wool next the skin' was good for the human body and so long-sleeved undervests and ankle-length underpants eventually became an essential part of the garments of even the lowest classes. The cult of allowing the sunlight on the body started in the second quarter of the 20th century and while men in Regency times would have worn a shirt and no underclothes, they always wore a shirt and would not have dreamed of working with a bare torso.

Bibliography to the appendix

Fashionable clothes in the 19th century... ... *Cunnington*

Occupational Costume ... ... *Catharine Lucas*

Lark Rise to Candleford ... ... *Flora Thompson*

A Country Camera ... ... *... Gordon Winter*

Old West Surrey ... ... *Gertrude Jeckyll*

The Costumes of Yorkshire. A series of plates published c.1830 (Possibly available in reference libraries)

Illustrations

Pages 1, 4, 14, 17 and 18
Courtesy of the Illustrated London News

Pages 2, 6, 12, 16, 20, 22, 23, 24, 25 and 27
Photographs and engravings from the Waterways Museum Collection, Stoke Bruerne

Pages 15 and 26
'The Quiver' 1897 (*pages 366–369 ' The Cry of the Canal Children' by T. Sparrow*)
Courtesy of Sally Hart

Page 11
W. H. Pyne's 'Microcosm' 1807
Courtesy of Luton Museum and Art Gallery

Pages 3, 8, 9, 10 and 34
Engravings from W. H. Pyne's 'Rustic Figures in a Landscape' 1827 and 'The Costume of Great Britain' 1805
Courtesy of the Kensington and Chelsea Library, London SW3

Pages 17 and 32
Photographs courtesy of Hugh McKnight

Page 24
Photograph courtesy of Mrs. Rose Whitlock/Robert Wilson Collection

Pages 28 and 29
Photographs courtesy of Harold Carter/Robert Wilson Collection

Cover and pages 5, 7, 13, 16, 19, 21, 24 and 28
Illustrations by Ann Aldred

Pages 30 and 31
Photographs by Derek Pratt

Costumes and photographs of canal life can be seen at the Waterways Museum, Stoke Bruerne, near Towcester, Northamptonshire.

Bibliography

The Waterways Museum – Handbook from Stoke Bruerne

The Microcosm of Pyne – first published in 1820

The Paintings of George Morland

The Paintings of John Constable
reproduced in various books on art.

Constable Country – James T. Pawsey
(*F. W. Pawsey & Sons, Ipswich 1970*)
Available from Colchester Museum.

Occupational Costume from the 14th Century to 1914
Phillis Cunnington and Catherine Lucas

Working Class Costume 1818 – Pamela Clabburn
(*Costume Society 1971.*)

The Railway Navvies – Terry Coleman (*Pelican 1970*)

Waterways Heritage – Peter Smith (*Luton Museum 1971*)

The Canal Age – Charles Hadfield
(*David and Charles, Pan Books 1968*)

Canal and Rivercraft in Pictures – Hugh McKnight
(*David and Charles 1969*)

The Vanishing Arts of a Peasantry – Camilla Doyle
(*Article published in the Burlington Magazine, October 1926*).

The Decorative Arts of the Mariner Ed. Gervis Frere Cook
(*published by Cassell 1966.*)

Our Canal Population—George Smith
(*Hodder & Stoughton 1877*)

Canal Adventures by Moonlight—George Smith
(*Hodder & Stoughton 1881*).

Narrow Boat – L. T. C. Rolt
(*published by Eyre Methuen 1944, reprinted 1957 and 1971*)

British Canals – Charles Hadfield
(*David and Charles*)

Occupational Costume – Moria Lister

The Number Ones – Robert Wilson.
(*Available from the Stoke Bruerne Museum*)

Household Words – Charles Dickens
(September 11th, 18th, 25th, 1858)

A Natural History of Man in Britain –
H. J. Fleure and M. Davies
(*published by Fontana 1971*)

Strata of Society – The Costume Society's Conference 1973